Gout Explained

Facts & Information

Gout Overview, Causes, Types, Management, Prevention, Treatments, Effects, Symptoms, Causes and Much More!

By Frederick Earlstein

Foreword

Gout is an arthritis that is caused by uric acid accumulation in the blood. This uric acid accumulation can cause sort of needle – like crystals that are usually found in the joints. This condition is very painful. If you or anybody you know has gout. Just ask how painful it is and I'm sure they won't even know where to start. It's extremely painful to the point that you won't be able to walk or it is even harder to just get up and stand.

When a patient is diagnosed with gout, what usually happens is that he/ she has elevated levels of uric acid. It can either be that the patient is producing too much uric acid in the body which is also something we will talk about later in this book as it can cause or trigger other health issues, or not excreting any of it in a normal way.

When it comes to the urine system, uric acid is considered as a type of waste products. Here's what is supposed to happen – the uric acid when it enters the blood should be filtered by the kidney (particularly the nephrons) and once done, you will excrete it in your body through your urine. This is why it is very important that uric acid is not lingering in the blood because if it does, the uric acid will transform into crystals that then goes to the joints. Like anything else, too much uric acid will somehow kill you through having a painful gout experience!

Table of Contents

Chapter One: What is Gout or Gouty Arthritis?

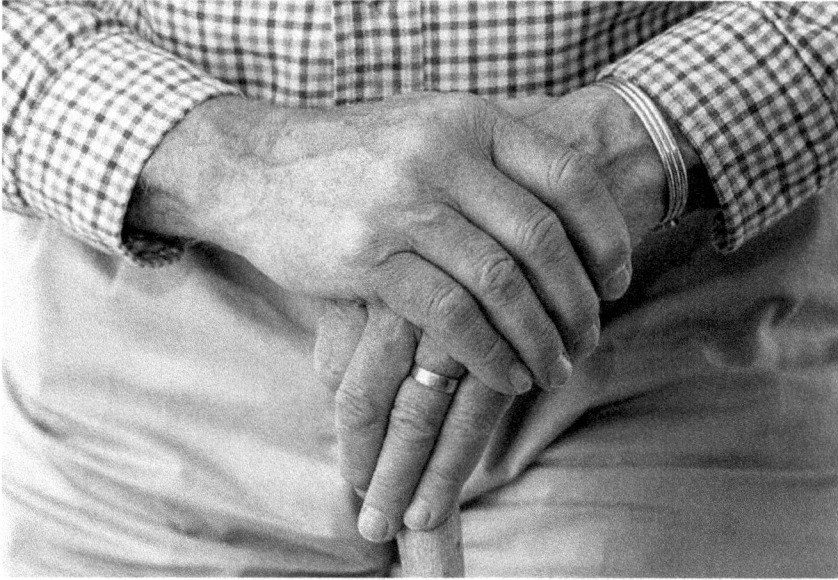

Gout is a disease that up until a couple of years ago had no new drug therapy for the last 40 years. Gout is something that most people don't think of it as a type of arthritis. There are over a hundred types of arthritis that we now know. Having gout is one of the best examples of an acute or inflammatory type of arthritis.

Historically, doctors treats patients suffering from a terrible pain of gout arthritis that's usually shown as having that swelling in the big toe; the patients will often feel relief after a day or two but as we now know today it is something that's chronic and that keeps coming back. Doctors now realized that having the acute gout attacks are just the tip of the iceberg, and that it should be considered something as a chronic disease just like other common chronic illnesses like diabetes or hypertension, which means continuous treatment and medication is needed.

What It Feels Like

The underlying problem with gout is high levels of uric acid in the blood. According to Sir Thomas Sydenham, an English physician, he described having gout as a person who went to bed in good health but suddenly woken up by extreme pain in the big toe, instep or ankle; and the pain feels a lot like a dislocation. A patient can't even bear the weight of the bed's linens nor the thought of a person walking in the room who can accidentally hit the site. The pain gets worse as the night goes on.

The situation above is exactly what happens to people experiencing a gout attack or gouty arthritis. Usually the gout attack happens early in the day and as the day progresses it just keeps getting worse to the point that the person can't even handle the pressure of the bed sheets brushing up their gout.

Renaissance of Gout

There's kind of a renaissance or a paradigm shift in the thinking of gout in the past two years, and that's because there's an increase incidence in certain populations and also the older populations. Doctors today have also learned to understand how the kidney handles uric acid and how it also plays a role in the gout problem.

Another important thing is the co – morbidities that comes along with gout that includes common illnesses like metabolic syndrome and diabetes, hypertension and dyslipidaemia, cardiovascular issues and age as well as obesity.

This is where most physicians think that there is a link between gout and cardiovascular disease because certainly these problems that were described are all major risk factors of heart disease. However, it is not yet accepted by all major health societies like the cardiologists or rheumatologists that hyperuricemia or gouty arthritis is a link to heart disease. But, there's a strong suspicion that in the future this can be proven significant.

Gout Stats

Just a couple of years ago, the incidence of gout in the U.S. was just about 6 million Americans but in 2018, a publication in a major medical journal showed that the incidence of gout affects 8.3 million Americans which is a huge increase in just a few years. If you compare these statistics to that of other related illnesses like back pain, fibromyalgia, carpal tunnel syndrome and rheumatoid arthritis, there's a significant higher number of patients suffering from gouty arthritis.

Important Factors to Remember

Gout is the most common acute monoarthritis or a single swollen joint particularly in males over 40 years old.

What's interesting is that women don't get the incidence of gout until after menopause, and the explanation for that is that the female estrogen helps lower uric acid in the urine. After menopause, the incidence of gout in women approaches that of men.

You need to also keep in mind that if you have concerns about gout, the solubility of urate is 6.8 mg/dl. So if a patient has high uric acid and therefore gout, and the uric acid is allowed to go above 6.8 then you can just assume that they are still depositing uric acid crystals in and around their joints. This could sometimes lead to inflammatory response or a chronic gouty attack.

Chapter Two: Progressive Chronic Disease

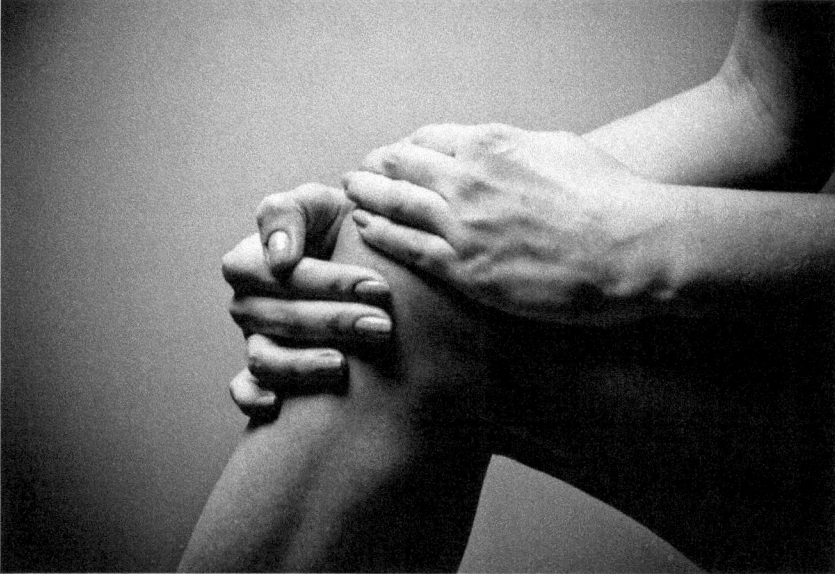

There's actually more people in the U.S. that has high uric acid without gout, and that number is about 32 million asymptomatic hyperuricemia. So if you have high uric acid, it doesn't necessarily mean that you have gout or that you will develop one, although it will increase your chances of it. So it all comes back to this link if there's a connection with diabetes, metabolic syndrome or cardiovascular disease. The first gout attack happens usually in the big toe but for some people, it happens in the heel, ankle or any other joints.

As the disease progresses, it characterized by inter – a clinical period, which is why it's suggested that there, could still be chronic inflammation even if you're not having gout attacks. And overtime if this is left untreated, patients may develop chronic tophaceous gout where there are lots deposits of uric acid in and around the joints. The most of what we're discussing here is microscopic wherein we really can't see it with the naked eye. But when patients develop tophi, they are large collections of uric acid that are visible.

In the scale of pain and time, what happens is that the patient could have a period of high uric acid and no attacks of gout, doctors refer to it as asymptomatic hyperuricemia. There's no evidence yet at this time that the patient has to be treated since there's no sign of pain. What eventually happens is that patients experience an acute gout attack. An acute gout attack can be resolved on its own, typically around 5 to 7 days. After that, the patient will experience no attacks of gout, and then the next one occurs. As time goes on, these attacks will become more severe and frequent especially if left untreated.

Uric Acid Levels

During a gout attack, the doctor will most likely check the blood work and uric acid levels but unfortunately, this is not the proper way to make a diagnosis, according to some experts. It is because about 50% of the time during an acute attack of gout, the uric acid level may well be low or normal. But that maybe part of the reason why some patients get acute attacks of gout – it's the fluctuating levels of uric acid. In fact, when physicians go to treat these high levels of uric acid, they may well precipitate an attack of gout.

There are really no normal values when it comes to uric acid levels. Obviously, if you've been diagnosed with gout, your doctor would want to keep your uric acid levels as low as possible.

In today's world with co – morbidities and medications that patients usually have to experience or take respectively, it's essential to understand that there are some drug therapies that can actually aggravate or worsen the condition particularly diuretics. Alcohol is also something that can worsen uric acid levels.

An example for a lab report of uric acid is this:

Suppose we have a male patient whose age is 50 years old. And let's say that his uric acid levels are 8.2. You will see in the reference range of lab reports (usually 4.0 – 8.5). So when you look at the range and the result of the example given above, you might think that it's still within normal and is of no concern but it really depends whether the patient has gout or not. If the patient as gout and the solubility should be less than 6.8 mg/dl then it means that the patient is still depositing uric acid around the joints. In our given example, even if the patient is within the range, it is still not less than or around the 6.8 levels.

The reference ranges used in laboratories have done thousands of tests of uric acid levels, and the 4.0 – 8.5 levels are the range where most patients fall but the real number to look out for is 6.8.

When physicians treat gout, their goal is to keep the uric acid levels not just within 6.8 but less than 6.0. They have to get the uric acid as low as possible.

Gout and Chronic Kidney Disease

A person that has been diagnosed with chronic renal failure or kidney failure (not necessarily people in dialysis) does complicate the management of gout and also some of the drug therapies that can be used. It also aggravates the uric acid level and leads to a high uric acid because the kidney is responsible for excreting uric acid. There's also good evidence that if one has mild kidney dysfunction or failure, that lowering uric acid can actually be of some benefit.

The medicines that are available to us, the Food and Drug Administration give us clear indications of how to use or why to use drugs. However, for rheumatologists and nephrologists, they think that for many of their patients, there is a benefit to not only monitoring their kidney function but also lowering their uric acid. Therefore because of these possible relationships with cardiovascular disease and the kidney, there's been evolving interest in the effects of urate and hypertension.

What About Diet?

Purines are breakdown products of protein. Protein can come from our diet or from the breakdown of cells in our body. These purines can be metabolize in the body into uric acid. If for instance, a person is placed in a healthy diet or the physician lessen purine intake, it can only result to a decrease of 1 mg/dl in serum uric acid which isn't huge. So that means that diet alone is not enough.

As far as diet is concern, there are few foods that people consume every day that contains high fructose or corn syrup. The worst are sodas and juice drinks. The dietary fructose or high levels of it can definitely increase uric acid levels.

Almost always gout patients resort to pharmacological intervention or drug therapies in addition to implementing a healthy diet and the likes. As mentioned earlier, we have new drugs today that aren't available back then which is an advantage for gout patients.

Acute Gout

75% of gout attacks happen in the big toe but 90% of the patients experience an attack in other areas at some other time. If your toe has sort of a lump then that's tophaes that was previously discussed; this means that there's a huge collection of uric acid in that area. On average, it takes about 10 years to develop but with drug therapy it can resolved although it won't happen overnight.

Now there are a couple of bodies or professional societies that established guidelines on how to make the diagnosis. In the U.S it's the American College of Rheumatology. One of the things they describe is typically a male patient who has acute gout arthritis in one joint particularly in the lower extremity, with tremendous inflammation. Sometimes the skin will peel like sunburn afterwards.

Some doctors try to experiment with it and try to get the fluid out; sometimes they find it but sometimes they don't. The fluid that comes from the gout or the swelling part is called monosodium urate crystals that can be taken from one patient's joint. There are times these joints produce sort of a white cheesy material that oozes out of the skin. It's so inflammatory and intense that if a patient went to the emergency room, the attending doctor might suspect infection but usually it's not infection, it's the intense inflammatory response of the body from the crystals.

Doctors usually get a sample of this for research purposes. It isthen observed in a so – called polarizing microscope. What they see is that the crystals usually appear very long and has some form of axis in it. It's usually colored yellow or blue depending on the axis. A physician can clearly look at the crystal and say, the patient has gouty arthritis.

There's another professional society that also established certain guidelines for the diagnosis of gouty arthritis and that's the European League Rheumatism. According to them, doctors don't have to stick a needle in every single joint. One can just look at the inflammation and judge it by the company that it keeps in like somehow who also has diabetes or high blood pressure, or someone who is older. You can also check it by also looking if the patient has high uric acid or perhaps have been diagnosed with heart or kidney problems. And through this, a physician can sort of make a presumptive diagnosis.

Radiographic Changes

As mentioned earlier, some people say they have a gout but what they don't realize is that there's so much more than just an acute inflammation or painful episode as it can be very destructive. If you look at the X- ray of a feet of someone who have had gouty arthritis, you will usually notice that the crystals or uric acid have somewhat destroy the bone in between the big toes and the feet. You may also see that the big toe loses a bone on top of it.

Gout can eventually destroy bones or caused well – punched out lesions as well as overarching bone. In addition to that, you'll also notice a density in the feet which is also known as the tophaes. These are just a couple of characteristics changes in the X – ray of a patient who has gouty arthritis.

One way for doctors to know if how severe or destructive a gout is in a patient is through seeing the radiographic changes as it can also determine what kind of treatment the patient needs. Some people even have to have amputations if it is that severe.

Chapter Three: Common Medications for Gout

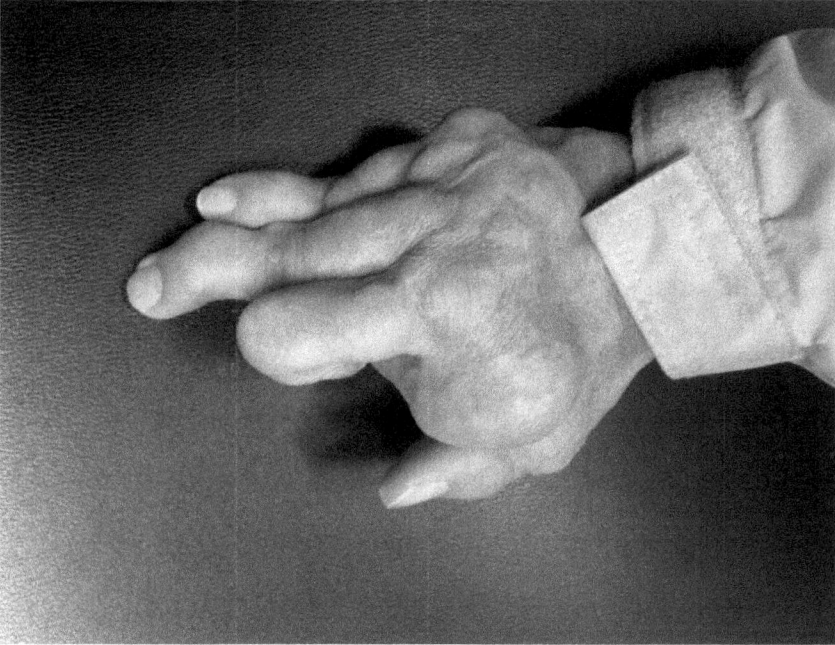

One of the first things that physicians do is to get over the acute flare, and depending on the doctor or how well – experience he/ she is, they often use anti – inflammatory. Your physician will prescribe the medication that they prefer. Usually the drug therapy depends on the co – morbidities so that it can prevent aggravation of other possible illnesses.

Other drugs include corticosteroids which can be injected or be administered by mouth. Sometimes doctors also prescribe non – steroidal inflammatory agents that are available over – the – counter. It also includes hundreds of drugs called colchicine.

Once the gouty attack or episode is over, the next step is to initiate therapy to lower uric acid. Now it can be argued that if patients only had one episode of gout, perhaps it's best to wait for the second episode to really be certain of the diagnosis. We can also argue that if you are sure the first – time, and crystals are formed then it should be treated as soon as possible since it's a kind of disease that can go on forever because it is chronic and incurable. The goal here is to reduce uric acid levels and reduce it below 6 as much as possible.

As mentioned earlier, when you lower uric acid levels, it may well precipitate an attack of goat. Some people or patience may interpret that as a failure of drug therapy but it's not because it's to be expected. We know now that at the same time doctors initiate medicine to lower uric acid, they also need to put their patients on something in order to prevent the attack of gout which could be anti –

inflammatory or colchicine.

The final treatment is to treat these people chronically. As mentioned earlier, doctors need to monitor and watch them over time; it needs to be treated over time and be considered as how one would treat patients with diabetes or chronic illnesses. They also need to check uric acid levels. However, if the patient or physician doesn't think about it, uric acid levels may not be routinely on the blood test which is why it should be kept in mind.

The other essential point is that prophylaxis probably needs to be kept for several months. Historically, people used to think that just a few weeks will be good, but what doctors know today is that it should be between 4 to 6 months.

Colchicine (Colcrys)

Colchicine actually has an interesting history because it has predated the FDA and it has been around for hundreds of years. But just in the past few years, this drug has become branded which is why it's also called colcrys. It's essential to do that because the drug – drug interaction and some of the toxicity as well as the appropriate way of drug dosage.

How colchicine works is quite complicated. When the crystal has gotten around the joints due to high uric acid, the white cells try to eat up the crystals. Colcrys has the ability to block the white cells who want to eat the crystals and therefore it can benefit inflammation. It can also block what the white cell produces which is called acydachine or a sort of chemical mediator. In addition to that, colcrys also has the ability to block the intake of these white cells and has also been shown to block the activity of the white cells.

Generally speaking, there's a lot of mechanism by which colcrys can benefit inflammation and gout patients.

Evidence for the Use of Concomitant Anti – Inflammatory Prophylaxis

As mentioned earlier, when it comes to starting a drug therapy in lowering uric acid, one should keep up the intake of colchicine for as long as 6 months. Again, it's not something that physicians have always done in the past. According to a small study, if the patient gets nothing (no colchicine intake), the patient can suffer about 4x as many attacks of gout compared to a patient who was given colchicine within the same period that they started the drug to lower uric acid.

When the experiment was taken out to 6 months further, the difference between the patients who didn't take colchicine versus to those who did is even greater. So what we know now is that a patient starts to lower uric acid, one needs a second medicine to lower gout attacks.

Colchicine Efficacy

According to another study about the pain score of patients taken in 24 hours after they had a gout attack. What researchers looked is the doses of colchicine (low doses compared to high doses compared to placebo). Physicians even today have been trained to give patients colchicine during an acute gout attack, one tablet every hour until they got sick.

If you take 6 tablets, the side effects may include diarrhea, nausea, severe cramps and vomiting but your gout will be doing great. Nowadays, doctors just recommend low doses like 3 doses rather than 6 doses. The pain response in 24 hours is just about the same in either group. There really is no reason to use this regime of one tablet every hour until you get sick.

Another study shows the adverse effects in the high dose group versus the low dose group. The patients that got high dose got severe diarrhea, the important thing is that the patient who got low dose, and remember they are painless and more controlled as the high dose group has low GI complaints which is why studies like this are important.

Colchicine Dosing

If you get gout attack, the recommendation of the doctor today, this two tablets of colchicine at the first sign of flare or symptoms and to take one tablet one hour later and do nothing for the next 24 hours and then start again with one tablet a day. For prophylaxis, if your doctor decides to start you on your uric acid as the lowering drug therapy, the recommendation is to take either one or two tablets a day for as long 4 to 6 months as previously mentioned.

Recurrent Gout Attacks

When it comes to incidence of recurrent gout attacks more than 1 year after each patient visit, according to a study from Japanese patients who have well – established gout and started drug therapy to lower uric acid; the lower their uric acid is, the fewer or less severe their gout attack. The incidence may somewhat be little to nothing.

There is a significant difference because if the patient's uric acid levels go just around 7.5 to 8, 60% of the patients will most likely have an attack of gout within a year. This particular study justified most rheumatologists that the goal is to not just get within the reference range but to keep uric acid levels less than 6.0 mg/dl as much as possible.

Febuxostat Efficacy

In the past few years, doctors learned a new drug medication or therapy to help lower uric acid known as Febuxostat with a branded name of Uloric. It went and passed through three clinical trials which is why it was approved.

The first one was a six - month trial, the second one was a one – year trial, and the last is for another six months. These trials compared Uloric acid (the new drug) to Allopurinol (the old drug to lower uric acid levels) which is what we've discussed earlier. What researchers did is that they measured uric acid levels of patients on a monthly basis.

What they found out is that in the first study of six months, 72% of the patients who are on Uloric were able to get to a lower uric acid level below 6.0 mg/dl whereas the Allopurinol group is only 39%. This suggests that the new drug is more effective than the old drug being prescribed. It doesn't mean however that Allopurinol is a bad drug; it's just that scientists found perhaps a better one.

In the one – year study, 74% of the patients on Uloric got to a uric acid level less than 6.0 whereas only 36% in the Allopurinol group.

And while researchers were conducting these studies and getting initial results, the FDA suggested to try it out in low doses. So in the last study that lasted for another six months, researchers included a 40 mg Uloric dose and found that it was comparable to the Allopurinol dose which is typically 300 mg per day. If you went to a higher dose, the Uloric drug will win again because most patients will lower their uric acid levels below 6.0.

New Drug Therapy: Pegloticase (Krystexxa)

Earlier, we discussed how Purines can be metabolize in order to lower urate or uric acid and that there are a number of enzymes in the body that help do that; this is how Uloric and Allopurinol work because they block these enzymes.

Unfortunately, for humans and most mammals, we don't have an enzyme built – in our bodies to breakdown uric acid into something that's fairly benign called Allantoin – some animals do and they just excrete it in their urine which is why they don't have gout attacks like humans. Just a couple of years ago, researchers came up with an enzyme to replace what humans don't have which is called Pegloticase (Krystexxa).

This is a phenomenal drug that can't make those tophaes we discussed earlier to disappear within 6 months.

Significant Reduction of Plasma Uric Acid

If you look at the uric acid levels that resulted from doctors' research, you'll learn that if patients receive nothing there's not much in effect but with Pegloticase (Krystexxa) it can be dropped to 47% in just six months. This is why it is a phenomenally strong drug but it still has some sets of problems or side effects.

Chapter Four: Causes of High Uric Acid

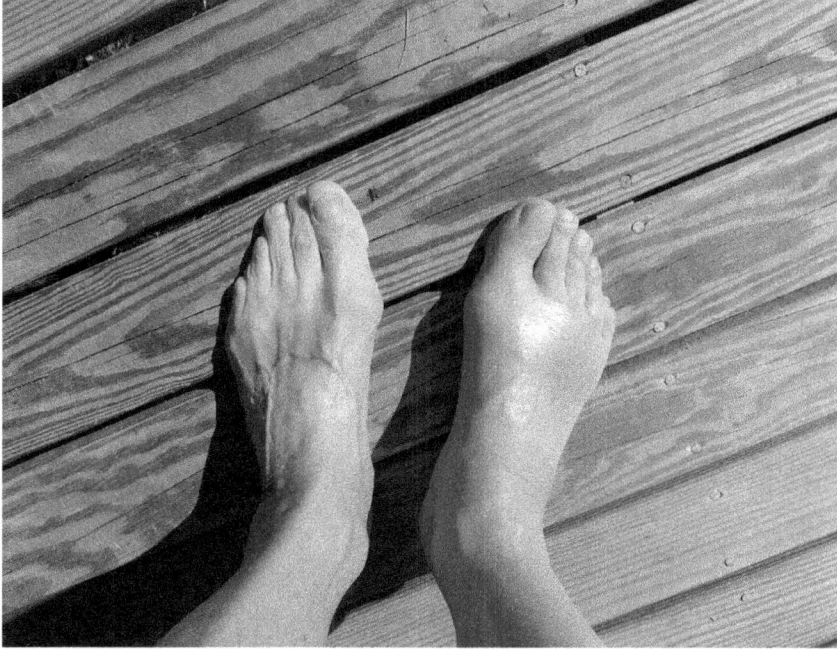

Uric acid comes out during the digestive process – it comes from what is called as Purine Breakdown. This means that uric acid is a by – product during the purine breakdown as your digestive system process the foods you eat.

Purine is a chemical compound used as a building block for nucleic acid (DNA or RNA). It can be found excessively in certain types of foods. If you are a nurse, you would most likely encounter purine being asked about in exams, especially the foods that are high in purine.

Causes of Increased Uric Acid Levels

Needless to say, if you want to avoid having too much uric acid, you should eat less of the following foods because they are simply rich in purine:

- **Internal Organ Meats** – this includes animal livers, kidneys and sweet breads. The sweet breads here pertains to other internal organs of animals like the pancreas or thymus that people eat especially as a street food.

- **Red Meats**

- **Seafood** – this includes sardines, tuna, anchovies, and scallops

- **Alcohol particularly beer**

In addition to what we mentioned earlier about high intake of foods that are rich in purine, other things that can cause it includes consuming high amounts of soda or fruit juice. These liquids usually contain high levels of fructose or corn syrup which are also shown to contain high levels of purine that can cause uric acid.

Alcohol is another thing that we mentioned earlier and how beer is also rich in purine. But when any type of alcohol enters the body, what happens is that it enters the blood and gets filtered by the kidneys and it then goes to the filtrate.

The alcohol and uric acid actually compete with one another to be filtered out. The kidney will choose the alcohol to be excreted in the body instead of the uric acid and leave the uric acid behind. This inevitably means that if you keep consuming alcohol, your kidney will just leave out the uric acid and it will pile up overtime in the blood until in forms into needle – like crystals which can then turn into gout.

Other things that can cause high levels of uric acid are kidney problems such as chronic renal failure. If the nephrons in the kidney which serves as the bodies filter are not properly working anymore then all sorts of problems can arise like gout or high uric acid. If a patient is diagnosed as chronic renal failure then it will have a hard time filtering and excreting body wastes such as uric acid.

Another thing that can cause high levels of uric acid is medications. This includes aspirin. Aspirin even in the lowest doses can cause high levels of uric acid. Another medication is called cyclosporine and diuretics. When a patient takes diuretics, the tendency is that they urinate a lot which means they are also at risk for dehydration. When one gets dehydrated, the urine becomes concentrated which is also a great condition for uric acid to build up or accumulate.

What a lot of people don't know is that diuretics medication has side effects and one of which is decreasing the nephrons' ability to excrete urea which is part of uric acid that can eventually cause high levels of uric acid.

Another factor is being overweight. If a person has a body mass index (BMI) greater than 25, they are at risk for gout as well. Helping someone or yourself lose weight by getting educated and putting in the work towards a healthier life can definitely decrease uric acid and therefore lessen episodes of gout.

Lastly is physical stress. This may include if the patient is being hospitalized and having an illness or surgery. There had been many patients who were admitted for surgery and have to come back because of complications and have somehow developed gout. Physical stress in the body can make gout attacks come out especially if they have a history of it.

Signs and Symptoms of Gout

Acute gout attacks tend to happen randomly. The person may have like a one – time gout attack in their lifetime or they may experience random episodes of gout attack which can tend to last 1 to 2 weeks. Between attacks that have more than one, they usually go around several months or even years because they experience another one. And since it is acute, it doesn't cause long – term joint damage compared to if the patient suffers from chronic gout attack.

With acute gout attacks, it usually starts with the big toe in the foot – the swelling of the big toe is a sign that uric acid is already at high levels. However, it can also found in the following:

- Fingers
- Elbow
- Wrist
- Kneels
- Heel
- Other Toes

What tends to happen is that it is going to come on all of a sudden and the patient is going to experience a severe pain and swelling of toes which usually wake them up at night. What happens is that the uric acid crystals have already formed in the joint/s. It then causes the joints to become inflamed including the surrounding tissue. This is the reason why the patient will often describe gout as having the feeling of a sand in between the joints and couldn't move it because it is extremely painful, which as you now know is uric acid build – up.

The pain tends to intensify within the next 24 hours. So you can expect that it is super painful but it will get worse as hours pass by. It usually peaks within 4 to 24 hours along with the stiffness. You might see that your big toe swell up and have some sort of protrusion coming out on the side due to inflammation of joints and have redness that's warm to the touch.

Here's the thing, make sure to not touch the swelled up toe or joints because it is very sensitive to pressure and can cause extreme pain. For some patients, even the bed sheet or the brushing of the linen against the gout can be so painful because that soft pressure can still intensify the pain, so make sure to not touch it. Make sure to protect the gout site.

Chronic Gout Attacks

Chronic gout attacks tend to happen due to chronic and elevated uric acid levels which then lead to repeated acute gout attacks. Whenever a patient has high uric acid levels, they will just constantly experience this acute gout attacks which can cause some issues to joints and bones. They will most likely have joint damage. From where those urate crystals form, what will happen is that they will get together and form large masses known as Tophi.

Tophis are white – yellowish nodules which can be found in certain places in the body – usually under the skin. It will be noticeable because you can see the yellowish or whitish circles in the skin. It is often found on the helix of the ear, elbows, fingers or toes. It can also be found on the joints and even in the bones. The large crystals that have formed together in clumps can definitely cause problems in bones and joints such as bone deformity and joint damage. The patient will also experience itching, acute attacks, inflammation of skin, peeling of skin etc. And since the person has high levels of uric acid, they are generally at risk of developing uric acid kidney stones.

Chapter Five: Inflammations of Joints

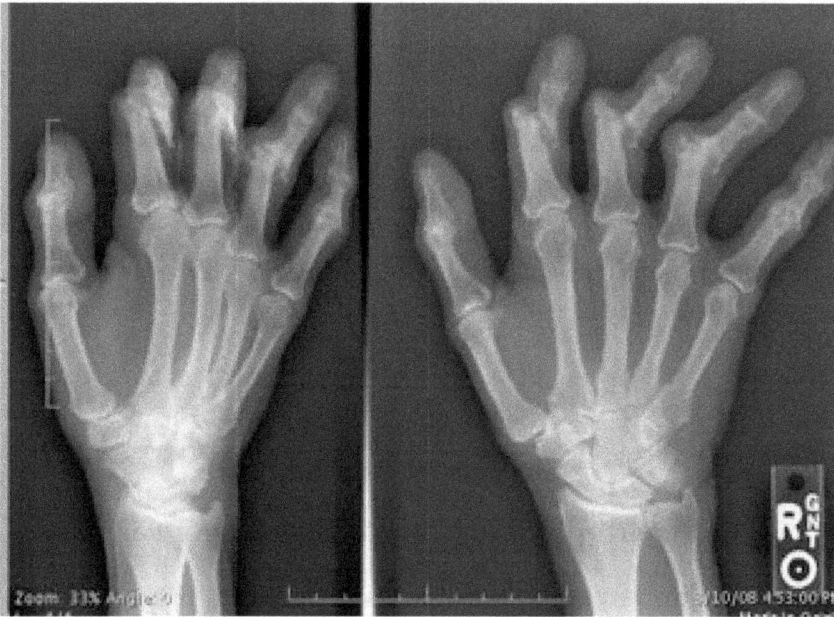

Inflammations of the joints occur in patients at the onset and the development of gouty arthritis. Inflammation is a process the body goes under wherein the body's white blood cells along with its immune protein assist in giving us protection from foreign elements such as viruses and bacteria. This is how our bodies help in shielding us from infections. However, in some diseases, the immune system of a person, or its defense system, sets off an inflammatory signal even when foreign substances are absent.

Conditions as these are called autoimmune diseases. This is when the immune system creates havoc over its own tissues responding as if healthy tissues were in a state of infection. Misdirected inflammation is the outcome of some types of arthritis like gouty arthritis, psoriatic arthritis, rheumatoid arthritis, and systemic lupus erythematosus.

Inflammatory Arthritis

Gouty arthritis is one sort of inflammatory arthritis that is accompanied by chronic joint swelling. It typically manifests on the joints of an arthritic patients hands, knees, feet, and hands. Arthritis generally affects the entire system impacting the body's organs. Patients who suffer from gouty arthritis experiences a myriad of physical symptoms such as swelling, redness, tenderness, warmth and stiffness of the patient's joints causing severe pain.

The motion and movability of the joints are compromised making the patient compensate on their movements by limping. More than one joint is usually involved. If left unchecked and untreated joints will begin to show deformity and the proper function and task of the joint/s diminishes.

Gouty arthritis is sometimes accompanied by fatigue, fever, and anemia. Fatigue is a common symptom of gouty arthritis and is most especially felt by the suffering patient when there is active inflammation of the joints. The body responds to the effects of the disease resulting in poor sleep quality brought about by pain. Fatigue is the body's way of reacting to the inflammation experienced by the patient's joints. It can also be brought about by the body's reaction to medication.

Because of the limited mobility and calculated movements of the patient, the fatigue an individual suffering from gouty arthritis can be overwhelming. This spirals to changes and sudden shifts in moods, relationships suffer, occupation and productivity is disrupted because the attention of the suffering patient is averted from the necessary task. Creativity can come to a standstill and the happiness quotient of the suffering patient is at a low. It is not unusual for those suffering from the ailment to display weight loss due to poor appetite.

Joints pains are apparent with people suffering from gouty arthritis. The joints of the suffering patient swell up when the disease is active and in full swing. It is not unusual for inflammation to also take place should the joints already have suffered previous damage. When gouty arthritis is active, it paves the way for the joints to swell up because of the lining tissue of the joint thickening and also to the excess joint fluid present in the localized area. When this transpires, the swollen joint expands and stretches out, irritating the capsule that encloses the joint. The capsules of our joints are fitted with nerve endings that send pain signals to the brain.

A patient previously diagnosed with gout can experience and suffer permanent deterioration of the joint, damaging the cartilage, ligaments and bones of the suffering individual - this will then cause extreme pain and utter discomfort when the joint needs to be utilized.

It is not uncommon for gouty arthritis to lead to tenderness experienced in the joints of the suffering patient.

The affected and inflamed joint lining tissue attacks and irritates the nerves in the joint capsule resulting in pain and tenderness. When this happens, the joint capsule is compressed by external pressure, and is felt through touch or when weight/ pressure is placed on the area. The pain felt is immediate and excruciating. Movement is not only limited because of the pain it is constrained as well because of the amount of pain and discomfort. This is why people suffering from gouty arthritis often, at the very least suffer from interrupted sleep and at its extreme, insomnia.

The joints affected by gouty arthritis become increasingly inflamed if not treated, and this leads up to the incomplete range of motion for the region affected. When loss of joint range of motion is present, weakness of the areas involved is reported. When left unchecked, undiagnosed and untreated, deterioration is inevitable and loss of range of mobility can become permanent.

Mild to Extreme Swollen Joints

Patients with gout have one thing in common and that would be the presence of swollen joints. The swelling of the joints can range from mild to extreme. People who suffer from gouty arthritis can usually tell when their joints are swollen because it is not only apparent through sight; it is also felt by the individual. When the joints of the gouty arthritis sufferer are in full swing, it makes it harder for the individual to move due to the loss of range of mobility on the affected area. Stiffness of the joints or difficulty in mobility and movement is another symptom of gouty arthritis. This is when the joints affected by active gouty arthritis are swollen and stiff.

Stiffness of the joint is usually more apparent and felt in the morning rather than any other time of the day. Physicians will inquire about the length of time the stiffness is felt by the patient, allowing them insight that gives clue to the gravity of the active joint inflammation. The duration of morning stiffness of the joints diminishes as the gouty arthritis responds to treatment given.

Redness and Warmth of Gout

Aside from the apparent swelling of the joints when the gouty arthritis is active, redness also is seen in the localized regions affected. The capillaries of the skin over the inflamed region widens due to the nearby inflamed joints of the area. The widened capillaries, also called dilated capillaries exacerbate the situation and display it apparent. When the affected joints of the patient are inflamed and the gouty arthritis is active, the joints are warm to the touch. Response to treatment usually addresses the joint warmth. There are cases and instances when there is no apparent redness or swelling, but warmth is felt in the localized region affected by gouty arthritis.

Gouty arthritis typically affects many small joints of the feet (the big toe) and fingers. It also typically affects the balls of the patient's feet. It is not uncommon to detect gouty arthritis to affect other parts of the patient's body like their knees and ankles. When this happens the affected areas become swollen, tender, warm and painful. The occurrence of more than four joints being affected is called polyarthritis. A few affected joints, when inflamed are called oligoarthritis and a singular inflamed joint is referred to as monoarthritis.

Bone Deformity

Chronic gouty arthritis can result to joint deformity in the suffering patient. When left unchecked and untreated, inflammation of the areas affected leads up to the deterioration of the cartilage and bone whilst loosening the ligament of the affected region. When left unchecked, permanent joint deformity and ruin will occur.

When it comes to limping, compromised lower extremity function due to gouty arthritis is made apparent by the patient's limited and labored mobility. Limping could be caused by a number of other ailments of the muscles, bones and nerves. However, in gouty arthritis affected individuals, the malaise targets the hips, knees, ankle or feet of the individual. A noticeable limp exhibited by the individual is caused by extreme pain and discomfort, a loss of range of motion of the affected areas, and is accompanied by swelling of the joint. Young children are not exempt from the symptoms of gouty arthritis.

Development Factors

The causes of arthritis and its development can stem from abnormal metabolism, infections, dysfunction in the immune system, past injury or the genetic makeup of the individual. In order to control pain improve and maintain the quality of life of the patient and to minimize damage in the joints, treatment will be needed. Treatment can involve physical therapy, 'patient education, and lifestyle changes along with administration of medications.

Of all the types of arthritis recognized, not one single cause can be pinpointed as the culprit as there are a variety of causes that contribute to the form and sort of arthritis a patient experiences. Some of the causes of arthritis may include abnormal metabolism which can lead to gout or pseudo - gout.

The genetic makeup of a person or a history of gouty arthritis in the family is also another factor that can be the reason of gouty arthritis in an individual. Injuries sustained, whether it is recent or long-standing is also a factor that contributes to the gouty arthritis of the individual. Lyme disease is one infection that can bring about arthritis. Almost all types of arthritis are associated to have a combination of all these factors. However there are some cases where there are no obvious or apparent reasons and which appear to be unpredictable in its occurrence.

In addition to the causes mentioned above, other reasons linked to the occurrence of gouty arthritis include the patient's genes to further increase their susceptibility and tendency to the risk of gouty arthritis. The diet of a person plays largely in the risk of developing gouty arthritis. Nutrition can also help in managing and avoiding the problems that come along with the occurrence of gouty arthritis in a person.

There are certain foods which provoke a negative response from the immune system which can make the symptoms of arthritis worse by increasing the likelihood of inflammation. Since gout is one sort of arthritis that is closely associated to the diet of a person, unhealthy eating habits can cause the uric acid levels of a person to become elevated.

Risk Factors

There are certain risk factors that are linked with gouty arthritis with some being modifiable while others are not. Age is one risk that increases the likelihood of arthritis as a person matures. Another factor contributing to the likelihood of gouty is the gender of the person. For instance, osteoarthritis is more commonly seen in females, with 60% of arthritis patients being women. On the other hand gout seems to be more common in men than it is in females.

There are specific genes that are linked to certain types of arthritis which elevate the risks of people who have history of the disease in their family. Other contributing factors of people who develop arthritis would be obesity and being overweight. Since excess weight is carried by the joints and bones of the body, the extra pressure put on the joints exacerbates the probability of gouty arthritis developing in a patient. To add to this, there are certain occupations that need to be carried out in a repetitive manner which can lead to the degeneration of protective cartilages.

Symptoms of Chronic Condition

The symptoms of the chronic condition are different from one person to the next and even the symptoms a person feels can change from one day to the next. These bouts of symptoms are what are commonly known and called as "flare ups" - when one or more of the symptoms are felt by the individual. When symptoms are absent, this period is known as a remission of the disorder.

Gouty arthritis is one sort of arthritis set of by an affected person's compromised immune system. This is when the immune system zeroes in on the protective lining of affected joints, causing a pronounced amount of pain that was otherwise not present before the development of the disease. Gouty arthritis affects the joints of the hands, wrists, the elbows, feet, ankles and knees of a person. It is also not unusual for the patient suffering from gouty arthritis to experience pain in the hips. When left untreated, the disease progresses cause a great deal of slow deterioration on the joints and bones of an affected patient.

Along with the damage caused to the vital parts of our joints and bones, which allow us mobility and movement, there are other, various symptoms that manifest it, marking the presence of gouty arthritis in a patient. Gouty arthritis is a chronic condition that has no known cure. Aside from damaging the joints and bones of an individual, it also affects the other systems in the human body. Getting checked as soon as possible is recommended since early detection, diagnosis and treatment increases the chances of being able to reduce the gravity of the symptoms, whilst preventing the condition from getting any worse.

It has been observed and noted that gouty arthritis is usually identified in adults between the ages of 30 to 50 years old. However, it is not uncommon for it to occur at any age, due to a myriad of reasons. The Arthritis Foundation approximates that there are at least 1.5 million people who have this disease with close to three times that number being women. Although a person who has a family history of gouty arthritis in their family would have a greater probability of inheriting the disease, people without history of the disease may also develop gouty arthritis. Patients with gouty arthritis may not immediately realize that they have the condition and the early onset of the symptoms may go unrecognized, or felt, for years. A person who appears healthy and mobile and active may only realize the condition upon reaching middle age.

Chapter Six: Early Indications of Gouty Arthritis

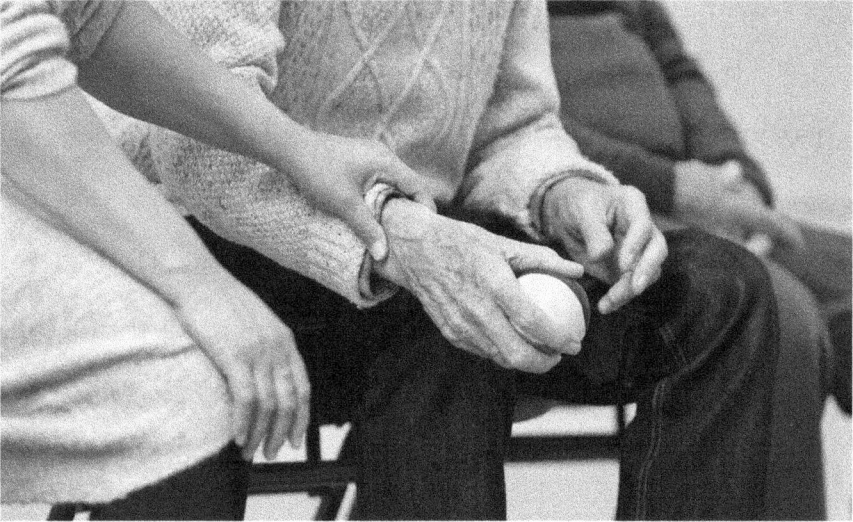

Most people with gouty arthritis are diagnosed when they reach middle age, but would have been experiencing the symptoms of the condition long before the actual diagnosis. The symptoms of early gouty arthritis largely go unnoticed because these early episodes happen occasionally and register mild and "insignificant". Other times, the symptoms mimic the symptoms of other conditions, like the flu. Talking about it with a friend who may be going through something similar doesn't help at all, because people don't exhibit the same sort of symptoms.

Symptoms of gouty arthritis are different in each person, so there is no way to compare or confirm the condition other than going to a physician where one can get a thorough check up and get a proper diagnosis. The experiences of one patient suffering from gouty arthritis can be totally different from, and not necessarily share the same symptoms with another person suffering from gouty arthritis.

These symptoms which fluctuate from one to the next sums up three characteristics of the condition; some people only experience the symptoms once and this may not happen again anytime between two to five years making the condition monocyclic. Fluctuating symptoms which seem to worsen then improve, experienced by other patients of the condition is called polycyclic. The third and most common of the characteristics of developing gouty arthritis presents itself and progresses to more severe manifestations over time. It does not wane and ebb but is constant. Should any of these symptoms be noticed by an individual, make an appointment with your doctor to determine if the symptoms are indeed gouty arthritis.

The signs of gouty arthritis can manifest itself such as one or more swollen fingers; one or more swollen knuckles; swelling of ankle or knee that last more than 6 weeks; swelling of elbow or shoulder lasting more than 6 weeks; having the sensation of walking on balls; fever and fatigue; flu - like symptoms; tiny, tender bumps beneath the epidermis of the elbow; stiffness in the joints of the wrists or elbows lasing for an hour or more during the morning.

Early Signs

Symptoms of gouty arthritis can start manifesting itself when a person is around 18 years old, and in most instances, the symptoms are more apparent in the smaller joints of the patient. The joints usually affected are those which connect the fingers to the hands and the feet to the toes. The symptoms are so mild that it is usually ignored and goes unnoticed. The pain that is felt by the patient may come and go; this is called a flare up. Flare ups are set off at certain times then completely fades away at other times. The experience lasts for more than a few days and can even extend for a longer period of time.

These signs include the swelling of the joints, tenderness on the joints when light pressure is applied on the area, feeling a warm sensation in the areas of the joints lasting for more than half an hour during the mornings. Other indications may not be as obvious and may imitate the symptoms for other medical conditions. Some patients develop low fever that cannot be explained away.

Then there are those who complain of feeling ill without an apparent obvious explanation or cause. There are also patients who experience a loss of appetite during the early stages of gouty arthritis leading to unintended weight loss.

In addition to joint pain and localized tenderness of the area affected, gouty arthritis symptoms become worse as the patient experiences chest pain, labored breathing, as if their breaths are constricted, the patient would also feel numbness and tingling. They experience utterly dry eyes, or in other patients, dry mouth. Patients would also notice red lumps that are painless in the knee region, toes or elbows. Patients may also suffer from anemia.

Complications

The early symptoms of gouty arthritis include anemia. Anemia is a condition when there is a lack of blood in one's system to supply the rest of the body. This happens when the bone marrow produces a low count of red blood cells than what is actually needed by the body. Red blood cells are responsible for distributing oxygen to the whole body and when fewer red blood cells are in circulation the body essentially lacks the oxygen it needs to use properly.

Anemia also is the reason why the bone marrow has lesser hemoglobin, which is the iron - laden protein, which is like vital oxygen to through the blood to the different parts of the body.

Various sorts of anemia are often related to gouty arthritis and these could include iron deficiency anemia and chronic inflammation due to anemia. The autoimmune response of a patient with gouty arthritis results to inflammation of the patient's tissue and joints. When chronic inflammation is active, it causes the bone marrow of the individual to produce lower levels of red blood cells, leading to the production and release of specific proteins which can affect the body in terms of how it uses iron.

Chronic inflammation can also disrupt the manner of how the body manufactures erythropoietin, which is the hormone responsible for and controls the production of red blood cells.

Some medications given to alleviate the pain and discomfort of gouty arthritis like non - steroidal anti - inflammatory medication can lead to the stomach developing bleeding ulcers. Medication such as naproxen, ibuprofen and meloxicam, when taken for prolonged pain management can lead to the digestive tract to bleed. This blood loss becomes a problem that results in the patient to suffer from anemia. If the anemia is too severe, blood transfusions are sometimes necessary to replace the lost blood.

Blood transfusions treatments will help increase not only the red blood cell count it will also elevate the iron levels. Aside from the fact that NSAID drugs causing bleeding in the stomach and digestive tract, these drugs can also cause damage to the liver of the patient. This happens when the food consumed by the individual is stored up and later on released for use. Apart from NSAID medications causing damage to the liver, disease modifying anti - rheumatic drugs, or DMARDs can also result to the same conditions of liver damage and anemia. A patient prescribed

NSAID or DMARDs drugs to manage gouty arthritis will have to undergo routine and intermittent blood tests in order to monitor the presence of anemia.

Anemia in a patient is not only determined through the reports of the patient, but is assisted by thorough check - ups along with vital exams and tests to make sure. A person suffering from anemia would complain of feeling fatigued and weak. They probably have difficulty breathing and would be experiencing shortness of breath. They appear to be pale and they have cold hands and feet. They experience bouts of headaches and chest pains due to the heart getting less oxygenated blood in the supply.

When a person complains of one or more of these conditions, the physician would order the patient to undergo a physical exam to determine if it is indeed anemia the patient is suffering from. It is procedural for the physician to use a stethoscope to listen to the patient's heart and lungs and inspect the abdomen of the patient by pressing on it so that they are able to feel the shape and size of the patient's spleen and liver. Blood tests are ordered by the doctor to make a proper diagnosis and these tests include a red blood cell count, a hemoglobin level exam, a reticulocyte count, a serum ferritin and serum iron. All these tests would determine the measure of new immature blood cells, the protein in the blood as well as the measure of iron in the blood.

Chapter Seven: Taking Care of Your Joints

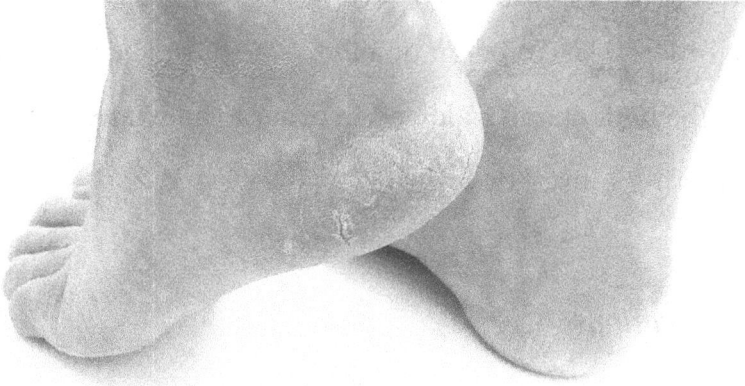

Just like the sole of your foot wear, the cartilage which acts as protective portions of the joints in our body also wear away with time. Without the proper protection and padding of the cartilage the bones will end up rubbing against each other which in turn causes massive pain and discomfort. The problem with a worn out cartilage is that once it is fed it does not here nor does it grow back.

And this is my arthritis is said to be a condition that has no known cure. Once it begins it is only a matter of time until degeneration takes place, therefore it is very important to realize how vital the function of the cartilage is to our joints and overall well - being. Knowing what steps to take in order to lead a better quality of life has to be undertaken by the patient and followed in order to alleviate pain and suffering caused by arthritis.

Medications

Over – the – counter painkillers can help manage the pain brought about by ice right this for short periods of time especially during flare ups. Some of the more common Pain relievers are ibuprofen, acetaminophen and Naproxen. These are good choices for short-term relief from arthritis pain however you should always consult with your doctor about the amount of pain relievers that you take and how often you should take them. Should you be taking them for a long period of time it may be necessary to talk about joint replacement surgery. You may also discuss Cortisone shots that could be helpful for short term flare ups.

Gout medications are recommended when it is tolerated by the individual however like most other medications in the market that is given to patients these drugs have potential side effects. Side effects may include allergic gouty symptoms such as diarrhea and nausea as well as abnormal blood counts and muscle weakness. Some medications can exacerbate and worsen the kidney stones while others can cause irritation of the stomach lining and develop ulcers in some patients.

Exercise Regimens

Stretching is a good way to keep a person, suffering from arthritis, flexible. Now only does it why flexible it also improves the patient's gouty arthritis range of motion and the way you can move your joints. This also is beneficial because it helps the patient decreased the odds of injuries and pain caused by arthritis.

Make sure that you always start your exercises and workouts with a five minute warm-up walk. After this you may lie on your back and stretch your hamstrings by looping a bitch around your phone using the sheet to help pull the leg straight up in the air. Hold this for at least 20 seconds then lower the leg you should take this twice on both legs. You may want to consider traditional Chinese medicine of acupuncture which involves insertion of find needles to certain target points on the body which can help alleviate pain and manage it.

Shed the Weight

Make it a point to shed pounds if you are overweight or obese. The extra weight that we carry puts a lot of pressure on the joints and on the protective cartilage that acts as padding between the joints. Losing weight will help take away the stress from your hips and knees. Every pound lost removes 4 pounds of pressure that is put on the knees that affects the patient.

Losing weight lessons the wear and tear in the joint and may actually slow the progress of arthritis. For every 10 pounds that is lost relief is felt because it will reduce the pain by at least 20%. Exercising is important in order to slow down the deterioration that is happening within the body and causing the pain of arthritis. The pain it still may make the individual hesitant to exercise and workout. But research has shown and proven that the stiffness and pain caused by arthritis only gets worse when a person is inactive.

Exercising regularly will get the heart pumping and will increase the blood flow in the body. Increased blood flow allows the cartilage to stay well - nourished and function properly. And as an extra benefit exercising helps the individual attain a healthy weight in order to keep in shape and manage the pain of arthritis. Staying as active as possible is very important make sure that your activity is something that is suited for you and approved by your doctor.

Avoid high impact activities such as running and jumping. It is best to choose exercises that are low impact like brisk walking cycling and swimming.

Possessing muscles that are strong around the joints can help the body take in some of the names that normally courses through the joint when in movement. Strong muscles have ability to absorb the shock that is normally felt by the joints. Ask your doctor or physical therapist what sort of workout you can do in order to build up the muscles that surround your joints doing so will improve the symptoms in your name and ankles. Only work with a personal trainer or physical therapist that has experience working with people who have arthritis.

Make it a point to stretch every day; stretching your body will help improve your mobility and your ability to move your joints without too much pain. Stretching not only towards of stiffness but it also assist in the protection of the cartilage from the normal wear and tear up every day activities. Some doctors recommend that their patience to Pilates or yoga in order for their patience to be more flexible. There is no need to attempt to be an expert in your yoga or Pilates classes,

Injuries

Whether you have sustained an injury from a recent accident or if you are suffering from any pain due to arthritis there are certain things that you should remember to avoid and so as not to encourage their albums or further the injury. There are also a few things that you should remember to do in order to manage your pain.

Continue with activity that you can tolerate and exercise as we quickly as you can. Cardio exercises are suggested in order to strengthen the muscles that carry the weight of your knees. Cardio exercises not only strengthen the muscles allowing for more confident movement it also increases your flexibility. In addition to these stretching, it's also very important to strengthen the muscles that surround the joints will not only allow you better mobility it will also curb the massive pain that patients who have arthritis endure.

When you experience any knee pain from an arthritis flare up or one that is caused by an injury, remember to give yourself a rest. You should then apply ice to the affected area so as to reduce swelling and inflammation. To prevent further pain, use a compression bandage and elevate the leg in order to recover from the flare up; if absolutely needed do not hesitate to use a cane, a crutch or a walking aid to take some of the stress off of the knee when in motion.

Aside from walking aids people with arthritis can also utilize gouty arthritis and splints to keep their balance while walking or when standing. When the knee is unstable or in pain, there is a higher likelihood for the person to fall and cause more damage to the knee area. Avoid these risks of falling by ensuring that your home is equipped with handles on staircases. If you need to reach for something that is situated at a high-level it is best to use a sturdy ladder or a footstool to help you do the job. Be sure to be mindful of your footwear as it can make matters worse. If you have osteoarthritis or any sorts of arthritis for that matter make sure that you use cushioned insoles so that it reduces the stress on your ball joints knees and hips.

A woman from any form of arthritis should try to avoid using high heels as these can exacerbate the condition. So best to find the proper insole for your footwear it is advise that you speak to a physical therapist or your specialist about what sort of insoles they recommend.

In the event of an injury use of cold pack to Isa swelling and to numb the pain of the injured area. You may utilize a frozen bag of peas or a bag filled with ice.

Apply it in soft cloth, ice pack to the localized affected area for about fifteen to twenty minutes three to four times each day. Switch it out by taking a warm bath or applying a warm towel or heating pad to the area for about 15 to 20 minutes as well 3 to 4 times daily in essence you want to alternate cold and hot compresses in order to ease the swelling.

Your doctor therapist and physical trainer will advise you against taking up any high impact exercises which can ensure you further and cause worst damage and pain. Jarring exercises including kickboxing, jumping rope, leaping from a high place, running, Lunges and deep squats are high impact exercises that create a lot of stress and put a lot of pressure on an individual's knees. Not only do these high impact exercises cause more stress to the knees were sent to pain it can also cause further injury.

The symptoms of arthritis are different in one person to the next. Each individual go through a variety of indications and symptoms that is not necessarily experienced by other arthritic patients. Therefore it is absolutely imperative that you had out and see a doctor in order to get properly tested and diagnosed. This will enable the doctor the recommend the proper medicine the correct exercise and any other walking aids that may be beneficial and helpful to the patient.

Eating Habits

Aside from giving advice to lose weight doctors will also investigate what sort of food a patient with rightists usually has. Diet plays a big factor in the development of arthritis in persons between the ages of 30 to 50 years old. Therefore indulging in foods that promote arthritis will need to be avoided in order to see the positive results of the treatment. Since gout is commonly linked with obesity, significant weight loss can improve the management of the condition domestically. Reducing calorie intake is a good way to shed pounds.

Doctors would usually recommend a diet that is low in saturated fat. They would normally recommend the replacement of refined carbohydrates like white bread potatoes and sugar with complex carbs like whole raisins and vegetables which help reduce the serum uric acid.

The doctor will strongly advise the patient to avoid frequent consumption of red meat and seafood. Avoidance of liquor and beer consumption will also be strongly recommended by the physician since alcoholic beverages increase the risk of gout. Aside from alcoholic beverages increasing the risk of a gallon sweetened beverages that is high in fructose corn syrup also heightens the possibility of the development of gout. And because that is a chronic condition if left untreated the patient may experience repeated painful and immobilizing acute flare ups of gout.

Complications of doubt may develop if it is not treated and eventual joint damage will be a parent and leave the patient immobilized with their quality of life compromised. Some of the risk factors of gout is hereditary and genetic and these make a predisposition for gout and preventable. However other risk factors can be curbed, like obesity diet and lifestyle

Chapter Eight: Alternative Natural Remedies

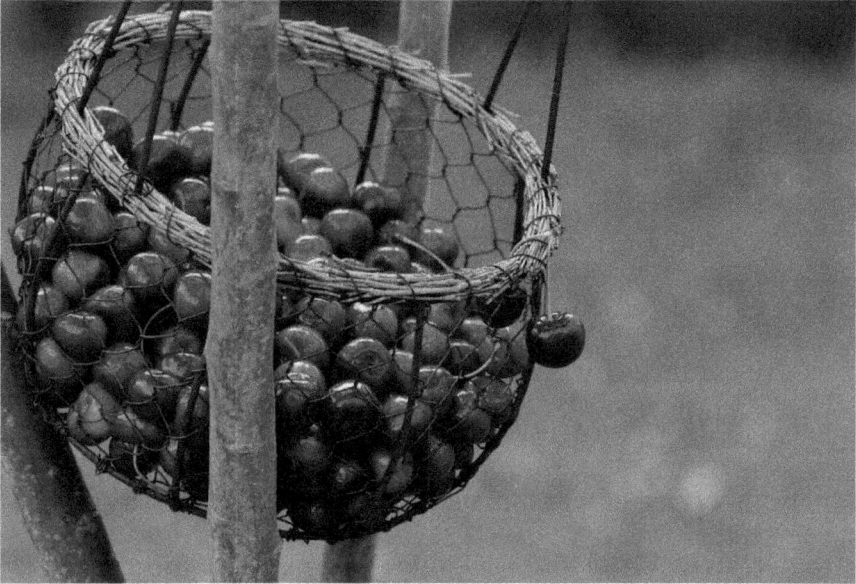

No matter how a patient ends up developing any form of arthritis, whether from injury or the extra pounds that puts pressure on the joints, or genetically passed on, all results are pretty much similar and unmistakable- pain and compromised movement as well as limited mobility and a shift in the quality of life are all some of the commonalities of arthritis in all patients. It is important that the patient experiencing pain due to gouty arthritis, see a doctor and get tested and properly diagnosed to get the proper treatment that they need.

If you are looking for ways to ease the pain and delay or avoid undergoing knee replacement surgery read up and find out about what you can do alternatively to taking over-the-counter or prescribed medication. The most common recommendation and medical advice that physicians would give patients who have osteoarthritis or gouty arthritis are to exercise. Inactivity does not help curb the pain that is brought about by arthritis. In fact extended or prolonged periods of rest can in fact make the condition worse and lead to depression due to the change experience by the individual.

Shedding extra weight is a heavy emphasis that doctors strongly suggest to their patients because regular exercise is one of the best way to not only get relief from the pain caused by arthritis it is also beneficial in terms of keeping the weight of the patient at bay so as not to put any more added pressure on the affected joints. Building and strengthening the muscles that surround the joints is also another method that works positively toward relieving and curbing the pain brought about by gouty arthritis.

Shedding just 5% of the body weight increases the patient's ability to move and makes a big impact on the reduction of pain.

Losing a more significant amount slows the process of the disease and this has shown positive effects and a better quality of life in the patients who have heeded to this medical advice. Physical exercise not only makes it easier for the person to lose weight it also allows the person to maintain a proper weight that is not a deterrent to their condition. The lack of exercise causes a domino effect due to the inactivity of the individual which can lead to weakened muscles increased pain less mobility and the worsening of the condition.

Physicians would typically recommend that you exercise so it is best to find an experienced physical trainer or therapist who can give you the best advice on what sort of exercises is good for you. Patients with arthritis are discouraged from taking part in rigorous high impact physical activity and are advised to take up low impact exercises, like yoga, tai-chi, Pilates.

Physical Therapy

With the help of a physical therapist you can work on targeting the weak spots that has been bothersome and painful and importantly can improve not only the balance but also the strength and joint alignment of the patient. Since other forms of arthritis has no known cure yet constant research is being done in order to provide more detailed guidance on how to treat people with arthritis even with gouty arthritis. And gouty arthritis patient has to take the responsibility of understanding their condition in order to avoid events that may cause further damage to their joints and most especially the cartilage.

Making it a point to build a strong understanding of how arthritis affects the body and the options available in terms of treatment and therapy is the best strategy for coping and managing arthritis. Learn more about the disease including things that you need to avoid doing so as not to worsen the condition.

Managing Gouty Arthritis

Many people who suffer from gouty arthritis are afraid to exercise because they think that putting added weight on their joints will worsen the condition when in fact knowing the rights of exercise that will help you will not only assist in slowing down the progress of the disease it will also give you a better mental outlook of positivity towards managing the disease.

You want to know what you are up against so that you know what to do and what to avoid. Some exercises can in fact cause more stress and more damage to the joints like the gouty arthritis pivoting moves during a football game or the movements carried out when skateboarding or downhill skiing. Understanding your physical limitations and sticking to a low impact program will greatly help you in managing

the condition without furthering the damage to the joints.
Do not attend exercise immediately if you have not at least
warmed up for five minutes by way of stretching.

Natural Remedies

More and more patients who have gouty arthritis are
looking to botanicals and herbs to help manage the
symptoms. Although medicine and medications have
changed the way in treating disorders such as this more and
more patients who have arthritis are looking to botanicals
and herbs to help manage the symptoms of gouty arthritis.
Many patients have chosen to explore another avenue of
pain management through substances derived from plants.

Consumer reports in the United States state that more
than half of adults in the United States take botanicals and
other natural remedies to prevent or treat disease. It is an
industry that takes in about $30 billion each year. A majority
of the people included in that demographic of patients who
suffer from arthritis. As with any other treatment for

whatever condition it is strongly advise that you consult with your doctor before taking any herbal remedies. And because arthritis is a disease that causes inflammation and joint dislocation as well as organ damage patients are never advised to rely on herbal remedies alone. Make sure that you consult with your doctor before you take any of the supplements in order for you to fully be aware of any potential implications to the medication prescribed to you and the possible side effects.

Botanicals come in many forms and in different varieties. The studies conducted on botanicals are commonly compared to standardize extracts that can be found in the form of pills there for utilizing other sorts may make it difficult The exact the proper amount as well as the active ingredient that the patient will be getting consult with your doctor and find an herbal specialist who has a track record of success in the field of botanical medicine.

Herbal remedies can be taken in infusions by adding the plant or herb to boiling water. These herbal remedies and botanicals could be in the form of flowers leaves, stems or roots. Some plants May only require just a few minutes of stepping in water whereas other plant products we require a longer amount of time for the active components to be released.

The most popular sort of botanicals sold is tea and it is one of the most well-known forms of herbal remedies. Tea is made through a process of infusion by adding boiling water dried plant products or fresh leaves roots stems are flowers. It requires just a few minutes of steeping. Mixture of herbal components and ingredients is called a concoction and can be prepared in several ways. It is usually prepared with heat. The process of adding a variety of plant products to boiling water like roots, berries or bark, is called decoction. When the preparation is complete the liquid derived from the decoction is drunk.

Liquid forms of botanical medicine, such as extract - drinks and oils are prepared made with water and alcohol. These are called tinctures. These extracts are created equal using a variety of solvents and liquids where in the liquid is allowed to evaporate in order to draw out a dry extract. Once the dry extract is complete they are formed into tablets or placed inside capsules and packaged. Extracts and tincture are more concentrated than herbs produced as tea. Lastly dried or fresh herbs are ingredients that can be grown or purchased.

Chapter Nine: Gout and Other Forms of Arthritis

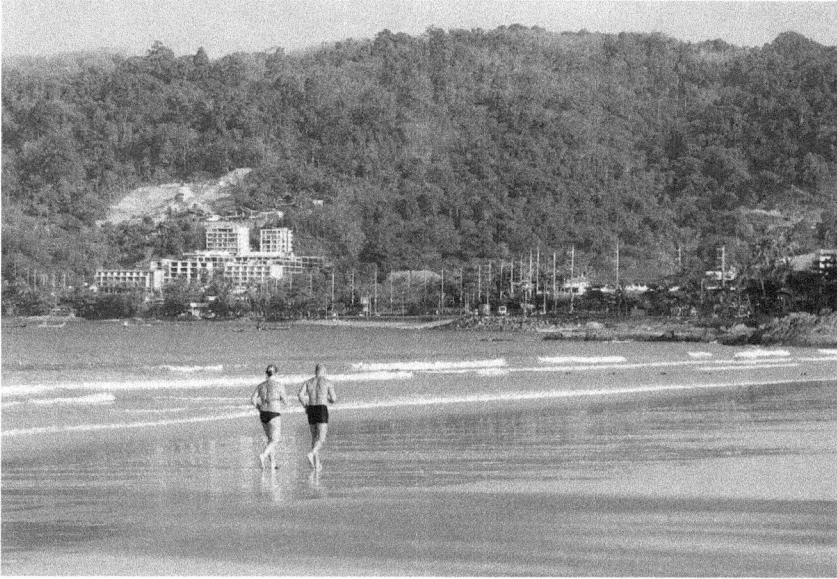

Gout is a sort of arthritis which results in a sudden swelling of affected joints. This condition is developed by uric acid crystals being deposited in the affected joint and can cause symptoms such as the appearance of nodules beneath the skin (tophi). A patient suffering from gouty arthritis would notice warmth, redness and swelling of the joints accompanied by joint pains. One effective manner of diagnosing the condition is for fluid to be extracted from the affected region and examined by use of a microscope to see if there is uric acid crystals present in the extracted fluid.

When gouty arthritis is left unchecked and undiagnosed, there is no way for proper treatment to be administered. If not diagnosed early and given proper medication and treatment, gouty arthritis can lead to irreversible damage to the affected joints, tophi and kidney damage, acute attacks of gouty can stem from dehydration, surgery, beverages high with sugar content or high fructose corn syrup. It can be triggered as well by alcoholic beverages such as beer, and other liquor. Gouty arthritis can also be triggered by consuming large and frequent amounts of red meat and seafood.

Patients who are diagnosed with gouty arthritis are strongly advised to change their diet and limit all foods and beverages that trigger the flare ups and swelling episodes that accompany the condition. Patients diagnosed with gouty arthritis are recommended to stay away from consuming too much fish, shellfish and seafood including sardines scallops mackerel anchovy codfish mussel's herring haddock and trout. Other meats such as bacon video turkey venison beef kidney Liver and sweetbreads are also to be avoided.

The signs and symptoms of gout typically affect one joint. The pain that the patient feels is usually very severe and is reflective of the Seriousness of the swelling in the joint. The affected area is tender and warm to the touch and there are some instances when even the slightest movement or brushing of object against it causes excruciating pain.

Joint effusion is the term to describe excessive fluid deposited in the affected area of the body. Gout usually affects the joints of the lower extremities of the patient's body usually are getting the big toe. This is a condition of gout the atrocities that is called podagra. However it is also not unusual for other parts like the photo knee ankle and elbow wrist hands and other joints of the body to be affected by gout. When gout is long-standing and severe it can affect multiple joints all at once causing joint stiffness and excruciating pain in multiple joints of the patient's body.

Gout can also be recognized through the presence of tophi. This is a hard nodule of uric acid that is concentrated under the localized affected area of the skin. It can show a parent in different regions of the patient's body typically on the patients elbow's on the upper ear cartilage or on other surface joints. When tophi nodules are present, these indicate that the level of uric acid in the bloodstream of the patient has been a high-level for a number of years. Went to fee is reasonable and apparent and medications and treatment is vital and necessary.

If left alone and untreated for a long period of time gout can lead up to physical deformity and joint damage especially trained physicians will need to employ the most reliable method to diagnose gout. They do this by extracting the fluid from the joint that has been inflamed and they test for the levels of uric acid crystals in order to determine if it is indeed gout.

The extracted fluid is then examined under a microscope in order to find out if uric acid crystals can be found in the specimen. This is an important test to carry out because there are other diseases and medical conditions like pseudogout which is a type of a arthritis brought about by the deposits of calcium Pyrophosphate crystals. The symptoms of pseudogout can have similarities that of gout. It is important for the patient to understand how a change in lifestyle can improve and greatly help in improving their condition and quality of life.

Limiting the consumption of foods mentioned above will not only help in preventing further damage it will also help in avoiding painful flare ups. Treatment and medication for gout typically fall into one of three categories; Prophylactic medications uric acid lowering medications, and rescue medications that give instant relief from the pain caused by gout.

When gout is uncomplicated infrequent and mild the condition can be treated with lifestyle changes and a change of diet. However even the most strict of diets does not decrease the serum uric acid well enough to control and manage severe gout. In this case medications are necessary to treat the condition. Frequent attacks that cost for uric acid kidney stones to occur and the presence of the fee or if joint damage from the gout attacks is evident medications need to be given in order to decrease the uric acid content in the blood level.

Drinking plenty of water for an acute gout attack can be a home remedy. If there are no contraindications such as lowered kidney function or stomach ulcers over-the-counter non - steroidal anti-inflammatory drugs such as ibuprofen and naproxen sodium can be taken by the patient in order to manage the pain. Keeping well hydrated by drinking plenty of water is beneficial to a patient in order to prevent gout attacks.

Rheumatoid Arthritis

This form of arthritis is classified as an autoimmune disease wherein the immune system of the individual suffering from the disease attacks parts of the body, zeroing in on the joints of the individual. When the immune systems attacks the joints, the affected joints of the patient become swollen and this can eventually lead to damage of the joints if left untreated. Rheumatoid nodules are bumps that develop on the skin of 1 out of 5 RA patients. These typically show up in the areas where the joints that handle pressure are located like the elbows, heels and knuckles of a person. Rheumatoid arthritis is a disease that still stumps doctors and specialists because they have not been able to figure out what causes the disease.

Experts are still divided on the causes of rheumatoid arthritis, with some supposing that the immune system becomes confused after a bout with infection, begins to attack the joints of the affected individual. This, when it happens, can spread to the rest of the body. On the other hand, researchers and scientists suppose that two chemicals in the body which are associated with inflammation - tumor necrosis factor (TNF) and interleukin-1, set off other components of the immune system. This being said, there are drugs that help block these chemicals from attacking the body, improving the symptoms of rheumatoid arthritis and preventing further joint damage.

The symptoms of rheumatoid arthritis are frequently more severe than that of osteoarthritis and the symptoms can suddenly show and feel apparent, or these symptoms can come slowly over time. Patients usually complain of stiffness and pain, reporting the sensation of their joints feeling "fused" together. The stiffness, swelling and pain is usually felt in the wrists and/or hands, the elbows and/or shoulders, the knees and/or ankles, the feet, jaw and/or neck of the patient. Rheumatoid arthritis usually affects more than one joint and is apparent in multiple joints of the suffering individual. The symmetrical pattern of the attacks of rheumatoid arthritis is common, meaning that if one side of the body experiences swelling and pain, the counterpart on the other side of the body will also experience the same.

Another indication of the disease, apart from the swelling and pain that come along with the condition, is the warm sensation felt in the area affected by rheumatoid arthritis. Swelling of the joints does not dissipate and can get in the way of usual daily and mundane tasks such as driving, walking, working, sweeping, standing, stooping, squatting (if you work on a garden). Even opening twist cap bottles and jars can be challenging for a person suffering from rheumatoid arthritis.

The sensation of feeling stiff would usually be the most pronounced during the morning, upon waking up and could last for the good part of the day, making it difficult for the patient suffering from it go about their usual chores and job. These patients would complain of fatigue and display a continued spell of a lack of appetite resulting in the patient's weight loss. Rheumatoid arthritis is opportunistic and could affect not only the joints of the individual; it can also have serious effects on the heart, lungs and eyes of the patient

Osteoarthritis

Another commonly reported form of arthritis suffered by people the world over is osteoarthritis and it affects millions. Osteoarthritis happens when the cartilage that protects and covers the ends of the bones erode and wear down over time. This condition can be present anywhere in the patient's body but is most commonly seen affecting the joints of the hands, knees, hips and spine.

The symptoms of this ailment can typically be managed effectively through treatment, therapy and medication (or the combination of two or all methods of management) but the process, once it has begun, is usually irreversible. Methods to manage the condition, and to assist in slowing down the progression of the disease, include staying physically active, regulating and maintaining appropriate weight (hence lessening the impacts on the affected areas), allowing for better joint function and lessening the chances of immobilizing pain.

The causes of osteoarthritis is the gradual deterioration of the cartilage which cushions the ends of the bones of the joints - when this happens both ends of the bones essentially meet and rubs up against each other therefore causing pain when or after you move. It is accompanied by tenderness in the region affected when light pressure is applied. You will notice a stiffness of the joints upon getting up in the morning or after a spell of inactivity. People who suffer from this disease find it difficult to move and get out of bed, especially after waking up. A grating sound or sensation when the bone is used is another strong indication of the degenerative disease.

Often times, the damage caused by the grating of the bones pave the way for the body to develop bone spurs to "compensate" for the gap. These feel like hard lumps which may develop around the joints affected by osteoporosis. When the cartilage, the firm and lubricated tissue which allows our joints frictionless motion and acts as a cushion that protects the ends of our bones in the joints slowly wears away, the affected joints rub grate against each other, signaling the brain and transmitting the message to pain receptors. The lubricated part of the surface of the cartilage then shows wear and becomes rough and infirm. When the wear down of the cartilage is complete the bone to bone rubbing makes for painful movement and limited mobility.

Research has shown that the risk of osteoarthritis heightens with the onset of age. As people mature and their bodies show wear and damage, the greater the risk. Though it is not clear why, it appears that more women than men are likelier to develop the disease.

The extra body weight of an individual can also be a reason of the wear down of cartilages. The more a person weighs, the higher the likelihood of the developing the disease since the extra weight gives additional stress to the joints which bears weight on the joints. The fat tissue then creates harmful proteins which cause the swelling in and around the joints of the area. When a person gets injured, whether from sports or an accident, the chances of osteoarthritis in that individual also increase. Past injuries that a patient may have healed from still and also make them a candidate for the disease.

Other considerations and risk factors that increase the chances of osteoarthritis in a person is their occupation. When a task requires a person to take repetitive stress on a particular and localized area of a joint, that joint may end up developing the disease. Even genetics is a factor in the risk of developing osteoarthritis. A person is more predisposed to developing the disease if it has been present in other family members. Osteoporosis has a way of finding its way down a family tree.

A person born with damaged cartilage or malformed joints are also more susceptible to osteoarthritis. When ignored and put off for later, this degenerative disease will worsen making it more difficult to manage; therefore it is important to get checked by a physician immediately. Severe pain can make even the most mundane of daily tasks, such as physically getting out of bed, difficult, painful and frustrating.

Early detection and diagnosis gives the patient a better chance of managing the disease, lifestyle changes, medication, and therapy can help. Symptoms of the disease usually develop gradually and worsen over time. Physical indications of osteoarthritis include pain in the joints while in motion or after movement. Tenderness of the joint affected is apparent when light pressure is applied to the area in question. Stiffness of the joint is most apparent upon waking in the morning; stiffness may also be apparent to the patient suffering from the disease after a period of inactivity. The loss of flexibility on the affected area is seen, and the full range of motion is depleted.

Another symptom of the disease is the grating sensation the patient reports when the joint is utilized. Bone spurs, or extra bone bits that form around the affected joints, feel like hard lumps. When these are felt and manifest in an individual it is strongly advised that the patient make an appointment to see the doctor.

Psoriatic Arthritis

Psoriasis arthritis limits the range of motion of the patient affected. They experience stiffness and tenderness of the joint. They experience bouts of pain caused by the condition. It is not uncommon for patients with psoriatic arthritis to notice their nails changing, an example would be pitting, and this is noticed in about 8-% of psoriatic arthritis patients. Roughly a third of patients suffering from psoriasis will most likely also develop psoriatic arthritis. The condition typically targets individuals between the ages of 30 to 50 years of age. However, it is not unusual to acquire the condition at any stage of life. This condition mainly affects the joints of the individual, causing the affected areas to become inflamed.

In order to determine if it is indeed psoriatic arthritis a person has, a doctor will have to order tests to prove its occurrence. Patients suffering from psoriatic arthritis would often notice swelling in their knees, feet, ankles, and hands.

It typically manifests itself through the joints causing them to swell. The joints would then get very painful and puffed up. The affected joints would feel hot to the touch and looks like angry red welts. The fingers and toes of a patient affected with psoriatic arthritis would puff up and look like swollen sausages.

Joints are painfully stiff in the morning making it difficult for the patient to move. It has a tendency to attack joints in pairs, mirroring the condition of one side of the body and expressing it on the other. It is typical to experience psoriatic arthritis in both knees, both ankles, both elbows and either side of the hips.

Stiffness and pain in the neck, the upper and lower back, as well as the buttocks may stem from the swelling in the joints of the spine and the hip bones of the patient, making movement and mobility painful and limited. Psoriatic arthritis is a rare disease as it is utterly damaging. The destruction caused by this form of arthritis quickly damages the joints of the patient at the tips of their toes and fingers rendering them useless. When this happens, and the joints cease to operate in the manner they are meant to, the patient can run into all sorts of challenges like keeping their balance. It would pose difficult for a person with deteriorated joints in their toes to stand or walk and it likely that a person suffering from psoriatic arthritis to have trouble utilizing their hands the way they are meant to be used.

The tendons of the psoriatic arthritis patient could also become affected through time. The muscle that connects to a bone could become inflamed causing pain with moving such as when needing to climb or alight stairs. Tiny dents and ridges, called pitting, are apparent on the nails of both hands and feet of the patient with psoriatic arthritis. The eyes too can become affected, making the colored portion of the eye; this can be very painful when exposed to bright light. Although rare, shortness of breath accompanied by chest pains can be some of the symptoms a patient with psoriatic arthritis feels. This happens when the chest wall and the cartilage joining your ribs to the breastbone becomes inflamed making it difficult to take easy breaths.

On even rarer occasions, the lungs or the aorta, which are the large blood vessel that exits the heart can be affected by psoriatic arthritis. Anyone diagnosed with psoriasis who experience painful hands will have to get seen by a physician immediately because of the higher likelihood of the patient developing psoriatic arthritis Patients may also get psoriatic arthritis even though they have not been diagnosed with psoriasis therefore any individual experiencing painful and/or swollen joint, irritated eyes and stiffness in the joints should head to see the doctor as soon as possible.

Early detection and an accurate and timely diagnosis of the condition will alleviate further damage and any deformity that would eventually prevent proper movement and ease of mobility. Expect the physician to give you a physical examination asking about symptoms you are feeling. The doctor will also be inquiring about your family's medical history as well as your own. You will be given a series of lab test in order for the doctor to get a better insight of what is happening inside of you.

Imaging, scanning and blood exams will help the doctor make a proper diagnosis. Because psoriatic arthritis looks a lot like rheumatoid arthritis, it will be likely that your physician will want to give additional tests to rule this out. The most telling indications of the disease are the skin and nail transformations that accompany psoriasis. Telling changes in one's X-rays will also give indication. A condition that usually rears around to ages of 30 to 50, psoriatic arthritis can also affect a young person.

Psoriatic arthritis can also manifest itself through red, itchy blotches on the skin. It also manifest on the skin as thick, gray, scale like protrusions. And because it can also affect the eyes of a person, there may be some swelling and redness that is apparent to a patient. Psoriatic arthritis and psoriasis are gene-related conditions that can be passed down from one generation to the next, therefore it is best to see a doctor when an individual notices or feels any of the symptoms that come along with the condition.

Chapter Ten: Summary

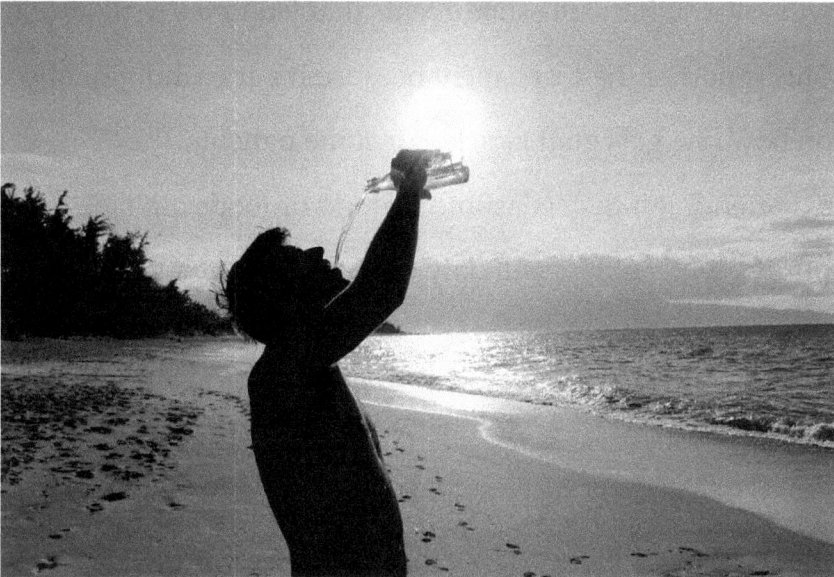

Here's what you can do if you suspect that you have gout; What you can do is to check if you have inflamed joints. You need to be able to assess it by looking at where it is located, the swelling, checking to see if it is red or warm, or how painful it is.

You also might want to check your health history because chances are you have experience gout before. Gout can also be developed along or be at high risk with other health issues like pneumonia or even just an infection.

If you have confirmed that it is gout, your physician will ask you if the possible events that led to the gout attack. This is part of the assessment because it varies individually on how one gets gout attack. For some patients, they experience it if they consume seafood or foods high in purine, while others will only experience gout attack when they become sick.

Your physician will likely educate you on the things you can consume. As mentioned earlier, it includes foods like seafood, internal organ meats, red meat, and alcohol especially beer because these have high purine. And then there's medications like aspirin, this is because anyone can buy it over – the – counter since it doesn't need prescription.

Usually, whenever a person feels pain, aspirin is the go – to medicine but what most didn't know is that, it makes their condition worse – gout wise since it increases uric acid levels. One should avoid fructose liquids like soda and fruit juice as well as avoid being dehydrated since all these factors can contribute to an increase level of uric acid.

If you go to the hospital, the nurse will most likely offer a cold/ warm compress for your gout if ever you can tolerate it. Another thing that you need to do is to stay hydrated; they would most likely advise you to consume 2 to 3 liters per day. The reason aside from keeping uric levels low is that since you already have gout, you are at risk of developing uric acid kidney stones. Keeping your kidneys flushed with water will keep those stones from forming.

You will also be advised to have a bed rest and cradle the affected part in order to protect the area with gout from linens getting on top of it or someone accidentally hitting it because it can give the patients extreme pain. If you are overweight, you can expect your doctor to educate you about the importance of losing weight as it can definitely prevent gout attacks from happening.

Medications

In this section, you will learn what medications your physician will order if you have gout. During an acute attack, you will need some form of relief since you will experience a lot of swelling and pain. Your doctor might prescribe you NSAIDs to decrease inflammation like Ibuprofen. They can also prescribe corticosteroids along with a drug called coldnicine.

Coldnicine prevent gout attacks and also provides relief due to ongoing pain and inflammation. It also decreases swelling and uric acid levels. However, the possible side effect is getting an upset stomach and also neutropenia which is decreasing white blood cells. You might easily get a sore throat or not healing from a wound since white blood cells are responsible for blood clot and helps the immune system.

Another side effect is also toxicity. The signs and symptoms of toxicity include numbness or tingling feelings in the toes and fingers as well as grayish colors in the lips. These are the things to watch out for when taking certain kinds of medications. Make sure to discuss this with your physician so that you would know what to expect and do once it arises.

You need to also make sure that you don't take the medications mentioned above with fruit juices or soda because it will increase the risk of toxicity in your body.

Another drug that your physician may prescribe is called Allopurinol (Zyloprim). This particular drug is used for the prevention of future gout attacks. So whenever you're having a chronic uric acid levels that are extremely high then your doctor will give you Allopurinol. However, it doesn't relieve current acute gout attacks so keep these things in mind.

Your physician might also advise you to get regular annual eye check-ups because such medications can cause vision changes. It is also best to avoid large doses of vitamin supplement while you are taking Allopurinol as it can increase the risk of developing renal problems.

Change of Lifestyle

Doctors encourage their gouty arthritis patients to change their lifestyle habits like cutting down on red meat, avoiding alcohol especially beer since it has stronger effect on the kidney compared to wine or other spirits, and how it handles uric acid. They also encourage and educate patients to lose weight and also limit high fructose corn syrup that we often acquire from drinking fruit juices or sodas.

Unproven Remedies

In most patients diagnosed with arthritis, or the conditions are chronic and incurable, it's been said that sometimes there's more money spent in unproven remedies than conventional drug therapies, and of course we're all aware of how expensive drugs are these days. The problem with unproven remedies is that there isn't always really good clinical evidence that proves that it's the right or wrong thing to do. There's always science behind it but always not enough. Sometimes unproven remedies cost way too much and sometimes they have patients avoid conventional care which is disappointing for most physicians as well as the patient because they thought they're going to get better but they don't.

One of the more common unproven remedies with gouty arthritis is the idea of eating cherries or black cherry juice. There are lots of patients today that consume large quantities of cherries, and according to doctors, there could be science to it in wherein there's antioxidant effect of cherries. But some people, they think that it's just good publicity for the cherry industry. At this point in time, it is still considered as an unproven remedy.

Putting It All Together

Gout is much more than that since it's a type of chronic progressive arthritis disease which is what doctors refer to as hyperuricemia. The target for most doctors is to make their patients' uric acid levels drop to 6.0 or less than with continuous monitoring. It's also best to be aware of concomitant meds that can prevent attacks of gout when therapy is initiated, and use various dose standards that we have in the past as far as we have a drug like colchicine and also be careful of other drugs that can aggravate co –

morbidities such as cardiovascular diseases, renal disease, diabetes etc.

Index

Photo Credits

Page 7 Photo by Stevepb via Pixabay.com,
https://pixabay.com/photos/hands-walking-stick-elderly-981400/

Page 12 Photo by handarmdoc via Flickr.com,
https://www.flickr.com/photos/handarmdoc/9209750197/

Page 22 Photo by handarmdoc via Flickr.com,
https://www.flickr.com/photos/handarmdoc/9212407896/

Page 32 Photo by cnick via Pixabay.com,
https://pixabay.com/photos/feet-gout-pain-foot-human-anomaly-174216/

Page 40 Photo by Esther Max via Flickr.com,
https://www.flickr.com/photos/esthermax/25251499775/

Page 54 Photo by StockSnap via Pixabay.com,

https://pixabay.com/photos/ball-people-old-elderly-man-2585603/

Page 63 Photo by congerdesign via Pixabay.com,

https://pixabay.com/photos/cherries-fruits-sweet-cherry-1503974/

Page 75 Photo by Em via Pixabay.com,
https://pixabay.com/photos/cornea-skin-foot-sole-of-the-foot-4418232/

Page 84 Photo by Qimono via Pixabay.com,

https://pixabay.com/photos/beach-running-old-couple-people-2090181/

Page 103 Photo by Olichel via Pixabay.com,

https://pixabay.com/photos/man-male-drinking-water-beach-937384/

References

Gout – MedicineNet.com

https://www.medicinenet.com/gout_gouty_arthritis/article.htm

What is Gout? – Arthritis.org

https://www.arthritis.org/about-arthritis/types/gout/what-is-gout.php

Gout – Mayoclinic.org

https://www.mayoclinic.org/diseases-conditions/gout/symptoms-causes/syc-20372897

Understanding Gout – Basics – WebMD.com

https://www.webmd.com/arthritis/understanding-gout-basic-information#1

Everything You Need to Know About Gout – Healthline.com

https://www.healthline.com/health/gout

What is Gout? – VersusArthritis.org

https://www.versusarthritis.org/about-arthritis/conditions/gout/

Gout – CDC.gov

https://www.cdc.gov/arthritis/basics/gout.html

Understanding Gout – Prevention **– WebMD.com**

https://www.webmd.com/arthritis/understanding-gout-prevention

Diagnosis and Treatment – *MayoClinic.org*

https://www.mayoclinic.org/diseases-conditions/gout/diagnosis-treatment/drc-20372903

Gout Treatment **– Arthritis.org**

https://www.arthritis.org/about-arthritis/types/gout/treatments/types.php

Sources of Arthritis Pain – Arthritis.org

https://www.arthritis.org/living-with-arthritis/pain-management/understanding/types-of-pain.php

Top 3 Types of Arthritis – WebMD.com

https://www.webmd.com/rheumatoid-arthritis/guide/most-common-arthritis-types#1

Understanding Arthritis -- Diagnosis & Treatment – WebMD.com

https://www.webmd.com/arthritis/understanding-arthritis-treatment#1

What Type of Arthritis Do You Have? – HealthLine.com

https://www.healthline.com/health/arthritis-types

About Arthritis – Arthritis.org

https://www.arthritis.org